Why He Stopped Calling:

Diagnose Why Men Grow Distant, Don't Commit, and Lose Interest

14 Ways To Never Chase Again

By Patrick King, Social Interaction Specialist and Dating Coach at
www.PatrickKingConsulting.com

Table of Contents

Why He Stopped Calling: Diagnose Why Men Grow Distant, Don't Commit, and Lose Interest
14 Ways To Never Chase Again

Table of Contents

Foreword by Gregg Michaelsen

Introduction

Are You Sure About This?

1. How To Never Chase

2. How To Create A Vacuum For Pursuit

3. How To Not Cling

4. How To Never Be A Doormat

5. How To Use Anticipation

6. How To Be The Prize

7. How To Not Mother And Nag

8. How To Seize Your Own Space

9. "So... What are we?"

10. How To Stay Independent And Yourself

11. How To Never Be Taken For Granted

12. How To be Confident

13. How To Make Him Feel Lucky

14. How To Be Vulnerable

Conclusion

The WOSR Cheat Sheet

Foreword by Gregg Michaelsen

I once had a client named Jessica reach out to me to ask the following,

> *"Why do guys love me for only a short time and then kick me to the curb? I'm a great all around catch! I go all in then always get dumped. Should I just give up?"*

It's a common question that requires a detailed response.

Jessica was a *yes woman*.

A *yes woman* ditches everything for a man that she wants. She compliments and fawns over him, and is at his doorstep thirty minutes upon receiving a text or call. Jessica thought that she was doing everything right and making herself irreplaceable to the man.

Her heart was in the right place and she didn't want to play games.

She was killing these guys with her kindness and generosity. In fact she was doing their laundry and even cooking for them without even being asked. And just two months later, you guessed it, she was single again.

Jessica needed help, and if you've ever found yourself in a situation where you feel like *you're doing everything right but getting the wrong results*, **Why He Stopped Calling** is the book for you.

My name is Gregg Michaelsen. I am dating coach for women in Boston and a #1 bestselling author. I have sold over 100,000 books in less than three years. Believe me when I say that Patrick has a unique way of showing women just how the male mind ticks.

Women like Jessica will learn exactly how to attract men while staying true to themselves. This book is the ultimate playbook and guide for women that don't want to play games to figure men out. Do yourself a favor and check out this book – Patrick won't disappoint.

Gregg Michaelsen *Dating Coach For Women and Bestselling Author*
www.WhoHoldsTheCardsNow.com

Introduction

You probably hear it all the time.

Your girlfriends (or perhaps you) constantly complain that the men they date treat them like trash and generally seem indifferent to their presence and affections.

That they are treated like a doormat, taken advantage of, and taken for granted.

Or that they constantly feel like they're the only ones that even care about the relationship.

Not to mention that the spark has disappeared and he's just not putting forth any effort in the relationship.

Is any of this starting to sound familiar?

So it was no surprise when my friend Victoria told me all of these things sobbing over the phone, wondering what she had done wrong. The answer was simple to me, and hopefully after this book it should be simple to you.

I told her that she had *ceased being herself*, the strong woman who had attracted her guy in the first place. She was a fiery, independent, occasionally aggressive woman that I could barely keep up with her in terms of varied interests. But after she started dating her guy, she turned, for lack of better word, docile. She started devoting all her time to him, and essentially quit her passions for him.

Why did he stop calling? Because she wasn't who he had gotten into a relationship with. There's a reaction for every action, after all.

Men disappearing, ghosting, or suddenly and strangely losing interest – your girlfriends (or you...) may actually be enabling these actions to a frightening degree. They might be the very cause of their problems, as Victoria was.

I've found that a large component of this problem is women operating on the mostly false assumption that men simply love women who take care of them. Sweet girls, girls who bake for them, and girls who "are fit to take home to their mothers."

This is true...

But ask yourself why *you* don't fall head over heels for a guy who loses all aspects of himself for you. Ask yourself why it gets old and why you start looking elsewhere for chemistry and a spark when that happens.

It completely ignores an essential component of what drives attraction in humans, both male and female: challenge.

People sometimes believe that the more agreeable and smooth a relationship is, the better. But that's simply not true, and results in a situation where women are constantly walked over and taken for granted.

There's a reason that so-called "bitches" are typically pretty successful in getting guys.

(The term "bitch" is used in this book not as a negative, derogatory slur for women – it's used as a descriptive term for women that simply aren't nice to others and let themselves be ruled by their insecurities, which creates an outward appearance of confidence.)

On the outside, they project confidence, have opinions, and aren't afraid to make them known. They are able to create chemistry because chemistry doesn't happen when you are just attempting to please someone. They are exciting, sometimes unreasonable, and unabashedly themselves. Sounds much more attractive than someone who simply says "yes" all the time.

Let's take a look at a man's inner dialogue, shall we?

Woman bends over backwards for him *"Hey, this is great! She's so thoughtful."*

Woman keeps bending over backwards for him *"Awesome... what a nice girl."*

Woman continues to subordinate herself to him *"...Again? Doesn't she have a life?"*

Now let's look at a man's inner dialogue when he encounters a **bitch**.

Woman sasses him *"She's got some personality! Definitely a fun girl, to say the very least."*

Woman calls him out on something *"Whoa, this hasn't happened before. I totally respect her more for it."*

Woman generally challenges what he says and calls him out on anything negative he does *"She just might be my match. I hope I can measure up to her!"*

You can choose to let someone have their way, or assert your needs as an equal priority. It's a very simple fork in the road that can either breed respect and confidence or being overlooked in the long-term.

You see, the issue with most men, and people in general, is that they fail to accurately identify what they want.

Men *love* nice girls. Who doesn't love surprise cookies and being taken care of? However, men do *not* love girls that cater to their every need and generally don't present any sort of challenge for them... or make him their first and second priority... or clings and suffocates like an omnipresent shadow. A *doormat*.

Men are looking for more out of a relationship than a caretaker, and that's what happens when you become too agreeable and sweet. The man begins to live in an echo chamber when you can never decide where you want to eat dinner. You create an unbalanced relationship is which doesn't give the man much else beyond companionship.

In short, men love bitches (on the outside).

It's easy to see the attractiveness of a woman who marches to her own drum, knows her self-worth, and can place other priorities above you. She makes you feel lucky to be with her because she's high-value and knows it.

Sometimes, just like male "assholes", these women can be flat-out terrible – where they treat men poorly because they can and don't care about them.

But there's an enormous middle ground between doormat and bitch – and that's what I want you to introduce you to. That's the zone of self-respect that embodies the great parts of the sweet, take-home-to-mother girl with the challenging and confident parts of the bitch.

And that's what this book is really about – becoming a healthy woman of self-respect (WOSR – this term will be used throughout the book!). You can give priority to your opinions without dominating others, and you can listen to others without becoming a door mat.

What lessons can you learn from the so-called bitch? You might be surprised.

In other words... how can you remain the quality, marriage-material girl that you are, but attract men with the bitchiest and baddest? How do you embody the traits that men think they want – a challenging, smart woman – and remove the negative implications?

You'll learn exactly how to walk that thin line like an expert in this book.

I'll break down the exact traits that cause men to flock to bitchy girls like moths to a porch light. On the flip side, I'll examine the exact traits that make women get categorized and cast aside as boring, unexciting *doormats*.

Learn how to transform your relationship into a true partnership by breeding respect and inspiring like no other.

Let's face what you've been in denial about all along – being called nice isn't a compliment. You can control your role in relationships and dating – what will it be? WOSR is the way to go.

Are You Sure About This?

This is a point worth repeating.

The typical perception is that a bitch is careless, indifferent, or loves jerking around the men that she is involved with.

Perhaps, but that's not what I'm proposing to teach you, nor am I saying that you should completely change your personality. That never bodes well.

My overarching point is that despite the overall negativity of a bitch, there are lessons we can learn from bitches in how they prioritize themselves and embody confidence. Combined with your own sensibilities, this will create the portrait of an incredibly well-balanced woman that can take charge in her relationships – the key to keeping a man attracted.

The intentions of a true bitch and a woman of self-respect (WOSR) are also vastly different.

When a true bitch outwardly manifests confidence or self-involvement, it's because she believes it will (1) attract men, or (2) successfully cover up her insecurities. Often, these are the women that proclaim that they don't need anyone and see everyone else as the problem in their relationships. She plays games and allows her insecurities to get in the way of vulnerability.

A WOSR – well, she comes with more self-respect, positivity, and true confidence in herself and her own self-worth. She places a high value on her own time, and becomes unavailable and aloof as a result of the dogged pursuit of her passions and hobbies. She also realizes that a relationship, important as it may be, doesn't define her or consume all of her time. She is her own woman.

The bitch doesn't text or pay much attention because she thinks that doing so will attract men, and she wants to minimize her chances of being rejected as much as possible. That, or she doesn't care about the feelings of the men she is involved with.

The WOSR will never overtext, and may sometimes be distant because she's so busy living life on her own terms.

It's a collection of personality traits and values that will offend and turn some off by their very nature... but the woman of self-respect is entirely comfortable with it. And of course, that kind of "who cares" attitude is *guaranteed* to be attractive to men.

I'm isolating traits that bitches display and turning them into assets for everyone else. It's okay to be a little more selfish and work on yourself, because that ultimately will pay dividends in dating and your self-confidence. In fact, the reason he stopped calling – counter intuitively, it might be because you are not being selfish enough. You're not being yourself anymore.

The rest is mother nature, as will be clearly illustrated through the following principles. After all, studies have shown that inconsistent rewards are addictive – isn't that exactly what bitches do, when broken down in the simplest of terms? You never know when they'll come through, so you are kept on your toes, and the anticipation has built such that when they actually do come through, it's a surprising, joyous occasion.

The WOSR promotes positive internal changes that result in an upgraded social and love life, while staying true to your roots.

1. How To Never Chase

Bringing him beers for when he watches football with the boys. Baking for him. Offering to pick up his dry-cleaning. Annual steak and BJ day: every day.

For some, that sounds like an ideal way for a woman to treat her man. Haven't we been forcefed the notion that women are caretakers, and should want to treat their men as best they can?

I for one think it would be wiser to use the money you'd spend on all of that on a nice mani-pedi for yourself.

Treat yourself as the number one priority and others will view you like that as well.

This isn't to say that you shouldn't make an effort to be sweet and impress a man that you are interested in. You should, and you should take care of your boyfriend or husband to express your feelings. But in the mix of dating, it's well-known human nature that when you chase someone too hard, it makes them far less interested in being caught.

It makes them bored. It repels them. Yes, taking care of them, mothering them, and generally doing too much for them – that's pursuit for all intents and purposes.

If you *overpursue* a man, it invites the perception that you have nothing better to do, that there are no other men that you're pursuing... and that you aren't a very high-value person in general. It's not sexy to tell a man *"I'm free Monday through Sunday, for breakfast, lunch, or dinner. Your pick!"*

You might even be seen as desperate. After all, doesn't a more charming and overall charismatic woman have men and people come to *her*? It's the epitome of the mindset of "If she's chasing me... she must not be worth it!"

We can debate the fairness of such labeling and perceptions all day long, and I'd agree with you that it's judgmental and ridiculous... but still stand my ground on the reality of it. There's a thin line to be tread, and you can either make a choice to play that game or decrease your chances of success substantially.

Pursuing hard also places you in the unenviable position of being labelled a "people pleaser," which is not typically used in a positive sense. People subconsciously lose respect for people pleasers and take them for granted, and you will be no exception.

The bitch never falls prey to this because she truly doesn't care about the man in question. She will never overpursue because she won't be interested enough to, therefore maintaining her mystique and allure. The bitch is confident (perhaps overly so) in herself, and assumes people will come to her. This brash confidence and mystique often does draw people to her.

It's human nature to be intrigued by someone that isn't intrigued or captivated by you, and again epitomizes another facet of human nature, "If you tell me I can't have it, then I want it even more!"

But what about the decent, sweet woman that enjoys being a sweetheart and basking in a man's presence and personality, and likes doing things for him, yet doesn't want to come off as overpursuing? How can she pursue him in an attractive, optimal way without overdoing it and *over*pursuing? How can the WOSR emerge here without playing games and manipulating how available she appears to be?

It's a mindset – one that will be emphasized repeatedly in this book.

You are a prize of a woman, and you shouldn't be compromising your dignity to pursue someone. How can you tell if your dignity is being compromised? Simply perform the "tell a friend" test. If you can tell a friend about your pursuit, and you get any negative reactions like eyerolls or groans, you've probably acted without dignity and not the way a WOSR would.

Repeat the following to yourself: this man, and everything that follows, does not dictate your life or actions. You have a strong sense of self. You are different from the rest of the women that will allow herself to be taken for granted, instead of demanding respect and yearning. A relationship is not your highest priority, and the alternative to being with someone – being alone – is equally acceptable to you.

In this mindset, you do not drop everything to pursue a man... you might not even drop anything.

Simply acknowledge your interest in him, and don't overdo it. A large part of why some women feel the need to overpursue and perform gestures is the insecurity that the man is not truly interested in them, so she needs to do all that she can to ensure that he is. You have to resist this urge because nothing you do inbetween actually spending time with him is going to tip the scales in your favor – it will likely do the opposite and disqualify you mentally. All you are doing is trying to create certainty in your mind, but that will backfire every time.

To the women who pay too much attention and feel the need to overpursue, I pose a question: Would you rather win him over or would you rather just satisfy your maternal sensibility and quell your insecurities? To win, you must leave him wanting more... which will cause him to want it all!

As I'll go over in depth later in this book, emotional uncertainty and a lack of sense of control are amazing aphrodisiacs. The bitch embraces this because she doesn't actually care about a man, and the man thus actually has no control.

The WOSR lives her own life... which keeps you in control and ultimately a challenge.

And who can resist a challenge?

2. How To Create A Vacuum For Pursuit

The mind has a funny way of playing tricks on us.

If something is less attainable to us, such as a jerk of a man who doesn't seem to care, they are automatically alluring and attractive for that very reason. We may not like to admit it, but someone of the opposite sex gains attractiveness points the moment they get into a relationship. The pull of the forbidden fruit is strong.

From the previous chapter, we learned that things that overpursue us are automatically repulsive and imply a lower value. This transfers to all walks of life — we have a tenfold desire for things we are told we can't have, and we never want something that is pushed on us.

Now here's a powerful trick that bitches have known all along and that everyone else should be utilizing: if you can subtly create a vacuum (a void where your presence and communications used to be — distancing yourself and making yourself more unavailable), that makes a man make more of an effort to be with you. It essentially makes him chase you, and eventually he will begin to believe his actions... and believe that you are worth the chase.

The bitch of course creates the vacuum by not actually caring about people and distancing herself.

If you as a WOSR create a vacuum and don't chase, you create the perception that you are otherwise busy, and don't or can't prioritize him. It's a fine line, but this perception is typically positive for you. It's what high-value people do in their daily lives.

When you create a vacuum, it is inevitable that he will seek to eliminate it by moving closer to you. He may wonder what you're doing with your time, think you're more attractive, or just plain be bored. Whatever the reason, there's going to be something niggling in his mind about you. Subsequently, when you stay still and he moves towards you, that's essentially him pursuing you. He probably won't even realize it, as the mind does the rest. Witness the inner monologue:

First: "Hey, I wonder what Steph's been up to lately?"

Then: "Say... I haven't seen Steph lately..."

More: "Is she ignoring me for another guy...?"

Finally: "Why didn't I ever date Steph...?"

The mind has a tendency to wander like a tumbleweed, and when you create a vacuum, the tumbleweed will inevitably drift to you and believe that there is a reason for that drift.

For example, what do you think about when you're dating a man? Probably him.

Just by virtue of having him on your mind so much, you are the de facto pursuer because you are oftentimes gameplanning your next move. Regardless of how much you like him, the man occupies a sizeable piece of your mental bandwidth for hours a week.

That's how you will occupy *his* mind and consciousness during a vacuum. He might even think that he caused the vacuum or is at fault for it, and seek to win you back and make amends. When you chase, sometimes you just want to win, and that's unrelated to the individual in question. This can work for you.

Creating a vacuum will also cause people to automatically respect you and defer to you more because they won't feel that they have the upper hand on you – which gives *you* the upper hand. When someone isn't present, we tend to forget the power imbalance that there might have previously been and are just grateful for their returning presence.

So how do you create the all-important vacuum with a man? How does the WOSR effectively use a vacuum to her advantage?

It's simple. Live your glorious life, and don't be available at his beck and call. In fact, sometimes make it a point to be scarce and absent. Don't manipulate your availability, but focus on your other priorities, and *demote him*. Don't accommodate him, or give in to your urges to see him or rekindle your friendship.

Chances are that if you're in love with a friend, the friendship itself isn't really based on anything real.

Don't reply immediately to him – because you're a busy woman! I would even go so far as to ignore and distance yourself from the object of your affection for a period of weeks to create the vacuum. You can then judge his interest level by whether he fills it at all.

If he seeks to fill the vacuum, don't cave immediately, even if you want to. As I will cover later, anticipation and the chase is one of the biggest aphrodisiacs known to man other than Marvin Gaye and oysters. After all, just because he has filled the vacuum doesn't mean that you give up your priorities.

Ultimately, people chase prizes.

By letting him close the distance and fill the vacuum, you have sneakily taken the place of the prize and object of his affection and goals – and he will believe that.

3. How To Not Cling

Pardon the imagery, but let's picture a bloodsucking parasitic leech for a moment.

A leech is completely dependent on a host body for sustenance, activity, and life. It will be drastically hurt if separated from from the host and generally cannot survive without it. We do not like leeches — actual leeches or the human equivalent.

When someone is overly dependent on us, every human has the immediate reaction of regret (buyer's remorse), wanting to withdraw, and general disgust. The first instinct is to create distance, not in a purposeful vacuum sort of way, and to seize their independence again.

That's because when someone is dependent on you, your independence is inextricably linked to theirs. They have just made you lose your own sense of independence. It hamstrings your sense of independence and imposes a burden of guilt and obligation that you haven't chosen for yourself. You can't in good conscience do anything you want when you know that someone is dependent on you and will potentially be hurt or distressed.

You didn't sign up for that!

Where is this analogy leading?

Being entirely dependent and clingy to a man like a leech will cause him to quickly lose respect for you and take you for granted. Who notices or cares about the shadow that is omnipresent? This book is about creating the most attractive version of yourself, and there is nothing attractive about a shadow that needs you to live.

This loss of respect and taking you for granted will inevitably set the tone for a relationship that will be unbalanced in every way... and you will be at the short end of the stick every time. Clinginess and dependence gives the man the pants to the relationship, the keys to the house, and ownership of that special pocket inside your pants.

About .0001% of the male population wants this kind of relationship dynamic with their significant other. Despite what you may have heard, it's not 1950 anymore, and men generally enjoy being challenged and stimulated... if not dominated occasionally. Changes are that you weren't clingy at the beginning of the relationship or when you started dating, so you morphed into a woman that was completely different from who he was initially attracted to. That's a recipe for disaster, and borderline unfair to him.

That is perhaps the encompassing issue with clinginess and dependence – it denotes a lack of strength that men innately seek in a mate. In other words, they don't want control of a relationship, and certainly not the total control that a dependent woman gives them. At best, it's tiring and annoying at times. At worst, it's an incredible turnoff.

Men want a partner and an equal. It's what they innately need, and thus is most attractive to them. Do you put yourself in that position or something subordinate and dependent?

Clinginess and dependence is undoubtedly the result of insecurity issues – you view the time you spend with him as linearly increasing the affection he has for you. So you keep doing it and try to bulletproof his affections. That's the opposite of attractive. To some degree, you need to let go and realize that that's not the person he signed up for and build confidence in the person that he did.

Guess what the bitch never does?

That's right, become dependent on others. This might be because she is too selfish or self-absorbed, but the bitch generally does not open herself up to the vulnerability of being dependent on someone else because she is scared of what may follow. The bitch keeps a healthy (or unhealthy) distance that appears mysterious and independent.

The WOSR dictates that her first priority is herself and her time.

When you value yourself and display your independence, men will follow suit. Think about the reason we all consider delaying replying to emails and texts — it's because we want to maintain an air of busyness and independence. We innately recognize the value of displaying our independence.

When you can create a lifestyle for yourself that truly is self-centered (and this term isn't used in a negative sense here!) and independent, you will also develop the strength men crave and seek out.

A huge aspect of chemistry is the concept of equality and meeting your match. When you have your strengths and he has his, the power balance is nearly equal and matches have been met — this leads to a great mutual respect. And with such a good balance, there is always an amount of uncertainty because you never quite feel like you have the upper hand, so there is always sexual tension, effort, and a subtle chase and dance.

Think about the conversations and sparks you would have if you met someone that could challenge you at your greatest talent. You may have started the courtship or relationship as equals or competitors, but somewhere along the way, you started to position yourself differently.

When the balance is tipped either way with someone being clingy and dependent, someone will become the reacher in the relationship, and someone will become the settler. Respect will wane. There will be a clear upper hand. This leads to a negative cycle of spurts of effort, and periods of complacency that plague all unhealthy relationships.

And guess where that ultimately ends?

4. How To Never Be A Doormat

Doormat.

It's a jarring term and one that men and women both treat like the plague.

It means that you as a woman have subordinated yourself to a man, regardless of whether you are benefitting from that relationship or not. You cater to his needs more than your own, and put him on a pedestal so high that you can't ever hope to climb it. Whatever opinion you have doesn't matter because his is more important, or you prefer to let him have his way every time.

What is central to being an unattractive doormat is the fact that you have lost your individuality, which has been demoted to a secondary priority. Obviously, this is insane, but it's not like doormats consciously make the choice to do this. It's a series of small decisions and concessions that lead one to the kingdom of the doormat – allow me to map the path.

First: "Sure, I'll come pick you up instead of having my monthly girls' night out!"

Next: "Don't worry about it, I was in the neighborhood anyway, here is dinner."

More: "Hey, I'm free anytime Monday to Friday, just let me know what works for you!"

Finally: "No, I totally understand, it was super last minute that your friend came into town so you had to cancel on me!"

If any of those statements look remotely familiar...

Oftentimes the doormat is borne out of an attempt to be overly-accommodating and not ruffle feathers. If you can make sure that you accommodate the man enough and make him supremely comfortable, he will find you most pleasing and attractive, right? Wrong. It's a fundamental misunderstanding of what men want in a woman, though sometimes it is hard to realize. If you hate it when a guy hangs around you and becomes your "yes man," the same is true when you become a "yes woman."

This chapter is about maintaining your independence and individuality outside of your significant other or woman that you are pursuing.

Let's take a look at our trusty bitch.

Maybe she's selfish, or maybe she just doesn't care that much about the men she's involved with. Maybe she is dating a few at once. Whatever the case, she keeps a healthy (or unhealthy!) separation from the man and keeps her own priorities as number one. She doesn't accommodate men and she isn't defined by her relationships with them. She may even actively rebel against them.

She will hang out with friends almost the same amount as when she is single as when she is with someone. What the bitch manifests as disinterest and lack of compassion, the WOSR manifests as a sense of strength and independence. You are not dependent on him, do not need him, and will be fine without him. Never let someone else define your world.

Just because he has injected passion into your life doesn't mean that he is the only thing you can be passionate about!

One of the biggest aspects of losing your individuality is that many women will slowly but surely stop standing up to or asserting themselves with men. They become okay with anything the man decides and are resigned to the decidedly dictatorial process they now reside under. It's a process that leads to being walked all over. As you can see from the above thought bubbles, sometimes it's so subtle that you don't even realize that it happens.

To expand on the bitch's mindset, your decisions shouldn't be based on whether they retain the man. You have your own principles that you should stay true to. You have dealbreakers and lines that shouldn't be crossed. If you constantly compromise your principles and identity for someone else, people will naturally begin to lose respect for you. If you back up and view yourself from someone else's perspective, you may lose respect for yourself as well.

Just ask yourself — would you make these concessions for a normal friend?

How many times have you heard anyone, woman or man, remark that they want someone that has their own passions and pursuits? If we trim away all the usual sunshine and rainbows attached to that statement, it really means at the root that they don't want to be the center of someone's universe. They don't want to be responsible for someone's happiness, sadness, highs, and lows.

It's a lot of pressure, and frankly, it gets old. It becomes a burden and takes away your independence and free will. What are they getting out of that relationship at that point? There's simply no incentive for them to stay with you.

People like to be prioritized, but when they are the number one priority at every waking moment, it becomes scary even for the most committed. For every dependent act you make, you inadvertently chain the other person to the label of "Jim AND Karen" which is cause for potential resentment and avoidance. They'll actively strive to be just "Jim" again.

Men want someone that can stand toe to toe with them because dating and relationships are about finding partners and companions, not "yes men" who give in constantly. Sometimes this means that arguments will end relationships or become more serious than they would have otherwise. This is not an entirely negative thing, because again... you do not need him, and you are your own strong individual. You shouldn't make your decisions based on the fear of a man leaving or growing disaffected with you. You become reactionary and aren't able to exercise your own free will.

When you are engaged in something, you become engaging – and being engaged in (or to) the other person doesn't count!

5. How To Use Anticipation

I'm a big hobbyist and believe strongly in pursuing as many hobbies and skills as possible.

My latest endeavor is painting, and it's truly been one of the biggest challenges of my life. I've always been good with my hands and have even done some forms of sketching and design in the past, but there is something about manipulating a paintbrush I just can't quite grasp.

And you know what? That makes me want to excel at it that much more, and I know that the ensuing victory will be that much more satisfying and triumphant than it would otherwise.

What does this have to do with bitches, WOSR, and becoming attractive to men?

The longer you have to wait for something you want, like mastering painting, the more you want it. This phenomenon of human desires transfers exactly to dating, courtship, and relationships. The payoff builds mentally along with the anticipation until someone reaches a boiling point and explodes.

The longer a man has to wait for someone he is interested in, the more he is going to want and appreciate her when he gets her. And if he doesn't get her, he will probably want her (you) even more!

If he has to work for it, wait, and pursue hard, it's clear that he is going to value it more than if you were supremely attached to him after just two dates. This isn't even bringing sex into the equation.

Of course, this is "the chase" that we all know and love or hate. There's a reason that many people look back on the chase phase as the best part of their relationships, and it certainly evokes powerful emotions. Everything is exciting and emotions are heightened.

In the context of this book, I'm defining the chase in the following manner: the gentle and delicate interplay between how much interest and reciprocation is allowed to be shown in a courtship.

Let's unpack that further.

The gentle and delicate interplay… it must be gentle and delicate because an unspoken rule of the game is that *you are not playing the game.* Bear with me. The aim is to make your lower level of interest and reciprocation appear natural, because if the other party figures out that you are indulging in the chase, it is automatically seen as *higher* interest and reciprocation. And you lose the chase.

Shake your head all you want, but embrace it. The uncertainty and lack of firm grasp on you creates anticipation and excitement.

How much interest and reciprocation is allowed to be shown... as I've discussed before, there is a delicate power balance involved in meeting your match. If you show too much interest, reciprocation, and *eagerness*, you run the risk of upsetting that balance and projecting the perception that you have lower value and aren't in demand. You have to be careful in how present and available you are.

Playing the chase correctly will create the anticipation of desiring something you can't have at the moment, but is close enough and plausible enough to keep you motivated and hungry for it. Studies have shown that inconsistent rewards are scientifically proven to motivate us more and evoke greater feelings of reward and satisfaction – apply this to your interactions with men.

The bitch keeps anticipation high by acting aloof and generally plays the chase excellently because she doesn't forecast or have much interest, if any. The

WOSR emulates those emotions by realizing that uncertainty is a powerful precursor to anticipation, which is a powerful driving force in human relationships.

Play your cards close to your chest and let the man drive himself crazy plotting his next move. The chase is only manipulative when you sit at home and plot how long to wait until you text someone back or how to avoid him. You're not doing this – you are making it so that you can barely fit him into your schedule and building anticipation naturally. After all, you aren't simply waiting at home scheming, are you?

As with before, keep your plans and activities for yourself. Keep your own priorities. Don't always pick up his calls or answer her texts in a timely manner. If he doesn't contact you at the proposed time, move on and make other plans.

Employ push and pull techniques where you show him attention in bursts when you're free, and zero attention when you're busy with other matters. There's no manipulation here – you're just doing what you can according to your busy social schedule.

If you stay in a perpetual chase phase by keeping anticipation high (and availability low) with any man you think that there is potential with, you build tension, attraction, and handily avoid the becoming a doormat and being branded as the "nice" girl.

6. How To Be The Prize

The dating world will always be unequal for many reasons.

Here's a dose of perspective from the male side: men have a more difficult time engaging with women and generally have a fraction of the options that an equally attractive woman might have. Think about it this way – when an attractive woman becomes single, how many of her friends suddenly turn into pursuers? Not nearly as many for a newly-single attractive man.

Therefore, men are generally more accepting of women that behave badly because their other option is to be alone. If a man doesn't proactively pursue women and isn't relatively handsome, it is highly likely that he will end up alone.

What would you say to a male friend that is being treated poorly by a woman? Something to the extent that they are too good for that kind of treatment and they need to find someone who appreciates them for them? Regardless of the circumstances or odds, this is true – people shouldn't allow themselves to be treated poorly out of desperation or fear.

Can you recognize this pattern in yourself as well?

It's not difficult to imagine that many women have also fallen into this trap. They've spotted a man that they are extremely intrigued by. He's handsome, high-value, confident, and charming. Women take whatever scraps of attention he throws her way because it's better than nothing at all.

We have become modern-day versions of Oliver Twist humbly begging for more soup.

Sometimes, we forget who we are ourselves – the prize. And we simply don't act the prize, so the opposite sex doesn't view us as one. We let our infatuations or other factors color our perspective such that the opposite sex is up on a pedestal and we are below.

My message in this chapter is simple – act the prize and men will begin to treat and view you like one.

The bitch acts the prize because she may genuinely think she is better than others and thus imposes that belief on others. She may not cause others to view her as such, but a little arrogance and overconfidence is decidedly more attractive than acting like you're grateful that a man gave you some attention. Her confidence is attractive and actually makes men think "Maybe she IS a prize!"

Have you ever been around someone with a low self-worth and sense of self? It's tiring because you have to be careful of what you say so as to not offend them and it tends to drag down the collective mood. It's just unattractive.

How exactly does a WOSR act the prize in a humble and unassuming way?

Acting the prize *isn't* about acting like you're all that and a bag of chips. It's a mindset.

A prize just acts like her time is precious and that people should be grateful for her presence. A prize isn't at anyone's beck and call, and certainly doesn't accept only scraps of attention that someone decides to give them. A prize takes pride in her own interests and zealously values her time.

A prize isn't a prize because she is above all others, she is a prize because she spends her time judiciously – and you may not make the cut.

As said before, if you believe yourself a prize (or at least fake it), others will follow your lead. The prize has more dignity and pride in herself than ancillary attention from a man can conquer.

A prize has confidence in herself and her capabilities, and doesn't let herself be disrespected or taken for granted. Confidence is a topic for an entire book by itself (and an entire chapter later), but is an amazing aphrodisiac in itself.

The important question herein is really whether others view you as a prize and how you must change that perception.

Here are some litmus questions to determine if you are viewed as a prize.

- How far ahead of time are plans made with you?
- Does he inquire about your schedule?
- Does he cancel on other people to see you?
- Does he apologize profusely when canceling and immediately try to reschedule?
- Does he present you with plans and options when setting up a date with you?
- Does he appear to have groomed or dressed especially nice for you?

Basically, does he treat seeing you as an important occasion?

Case in point - booty calls are great. However, booty calls are sometimes motivated by emotions that aren't the most positive despite the benefits you might be getting. Don't mistake his contacting you as spontaneous longing. You might just be convenient, and he might just be passing time. Does a prize become a booty call?

If you're getting a call at 2:00 AM, you can feel free to cheer and start cleaning your room, but I propose that you should think about exactly why the call came so late. Namely, that you are the backup for the night, and are better company than no one at all – not quite a prize, is it? A WOSR might just turn her phone on silent and go back to sleep rather than entertain dubious attention from a dubious source. She's better than that and doesn't need it.

So if you really value cultivating your image as a prize, resist answering that call, no matter how much you want to hitch the train to sex town. You will drastically change the perception of power in that relationship, and make yourself a challenge that he must conquer.

A prize doesn't accept being treated like a backup. If someone doesn't hold you in the regard of a prize, why do you want to be with someone like that... or in a relationship that is already so unbalanced and skewed towards satisfying only him? Would you accept that kind of treatment from a normal friend?

A prize doesn't apologize to men purely out of instinct and to avoid conflict; she requires a clear reason because a prize knows her worth and doesn't pander to others. If he asks how your schedule is the next week, give only a couple of specific openings, because a prize is constantly keeps himself busy and fills her schedule quickly. A prize doesn't accept poor treatment from men and will show displeasure accordingly.

This process begins within. When you clearly treat yourself like a priority, others will take notice and follow. A prize doesn't make decisions based on fear.

7. How To Not Mother And Nag

Whether you realize it or not, gender roles still play a large part in our society.

Males certainly feel the pressure to be the breadwinners in most traditional settings, and women in turn feel the pressure (both internal and external) to be the nurturers, caretakers, and outward manifestation of the maternal instinct.

These gender roles are in a sense, directly tied to our modern day conception of romance. Chivalry? The Damsel in distress? The Caretaker. The Defender. And so on.

However, all of those roles are predicated on treating your man in the primal way that a woman does for his mate... and not in the way that a mother takes care of her son. There's a big difference, but it's easy to cross over. Your interactions must straddle the sometimes thin line between your nurturing instincts and smothering mother territory.

It is imperative that you do not mother – he already has one and doesn't need an additional source of nagging, especially not from the person that should ideally be an equal partner and sexual mate. See how the roles are being weirdly blurred already?

Mothering has the distinct effect of making someone feel smothered and that they are being tracked by someone for their own purposes – not that they are being taken care of and treated like an independent man. It's annoying and almost always a negative statement at something they can improve on.

It makes people feel cornered and defensive instantly instead of thankful and aroused.

For those of you that did not have overbearing mothers or fathers growing up, here's what mothers do: ask you where you were, ask you to check in with them, account for time away from them, be overly clingy and focused on you, place their own expectations on you, be preachy about what you're doing and who you're seeing, dote too much, and assume that will be spent together.

Now that we're all working within the same context – how does someone like that make you feel? Especially someone that is supposed to be your mate and partner?

Annoyed, smothered, mothered, and ultimately wanting to break free and get away. "Whew, thank God I got away from him for the night! She's TOO much!" Yup, you're creating the same effect in a man when you treat them like a son/inmate and not like a mate. You're also subtly beating down their sense of self-esteem because you are implying or outright saying that they are not keeping in line with your expectations of them.

Some men ultimately come to the conclusion that they want to marry someone very similar to their mother – but absolutely not in this aspect. They spent (around) eighteen years living under the same roof with them and taking orders from them already, they don't want any more!

You will create the same instinct that a man will feel if you overly dote and become dependent and clingy on him. He'll feel cornered and instantly look for an escape route… and by creating that distance, it instantly turns you into the pursuer. We've gone over why this is a losing proposition for you.

He might even lash out against you as a son would to his mother setting her curfew. Then it's up to you to pick up the pieces and go after him and apologize – a pattern which might be doomed to repeat itself over and over again.

Finally, men don't often have romantic chemistry with their mothers or anyone that they feel is nagging and watching them like a hawk. The day to day relationship you will create is a cycle of nagging, arguing, caretaking, and acceptance. Sexual chemistry and desire don't belong in that cycle whatsoever – resentment is far more common.

Even if he likes you and doesn't mind the excessive amount of attention and oversight, you create a negative association with each of your interactions – he will feel obligated to spend time with you and may even do so out of guilt. You're putting your expectations on someone else, and anytime that happens, they will feel burdened to have to live up to them.

Is it positive to have someone spend time with you out of a feeling of duty or guilt? Of course not! Your time spent together and dates should be highly anticipated and looked forward to.

A bitch probably doesn't have a mothering problem because she doesn't care about the well-being of the men that she dates. This preserves her mental space for sexual chemistry and desire, which is a benefit of that otherwise negative approach.

How does the WOSR treat her man as a mate and not as a son? She takes care of him, but doesn't nag that everything is in order. The WOSR can take care of herself and assumes that her man can as well. It's up to him to change things himself if he deems it necessary, and you can't be the one driving his life along for him.

She doesn't do things that a mother would and shows her affections in ways that are romantic as opposed to serving. You might think that your attention to his outfit is caring, but is it serving or romantic?

Your focus should be on romantic gestures that a mate uses for seduction, and not overbearing mother gestures that will drive him to rebel against you. Contact him to demonstrate that you miss him, but not to make sure that he's okay, had his vitamins, and hear about every detail. Buy him a new outfit because it makes you hot to see him in it, not because he needs new jeans desperately. Ask him to do the dishes because you love a man who is industrious.

Generally speaking, mothering is an instinct that is somewhat selfish. You mother him because something bothers you, not him – and it benefits you, not him. If you find that is your motivation, you need to take a step back and realize how that positions you in the relationship.

8. How To Seize Your Own Space

There's a saying that goes "If you love someone, set them free... and if they return to you, then it was meant to be."

Of course, it's bullshit. If you want that to happen in real life, you should just buy a boomerang.

Giving someone space is when you remain in the same proximity, but allow someone else to have freedom and not be obligated to you. It sounds generous and something that a trustworthy woman would do, but it can often backfire on you.

If you give someone the space they want, they'll almost never look back to you. The saying mostly gives people a hopeful silver lining in the context of a breakup.

Giving someone else space is backing off and giving them free reign. Space, when given to others like a release from jail, is not going to help you. But when you cleverly give *yourself* space, that void will only serve to draw men to you.

In other words, when you give men too much space and time to themselves, it's not a guarantee that they'll come back to you... they may run from you, get bored, or get distracted by the next shiny object that comes along– further, this takes matters out of your hands, which is never the goal. You want to be an independent WOSR, but you still need to be a presence in their lives.

For example, giving a man the freedom to speak and flirt with other women is something that can be seen as gifting space. But it can backfire and may achieve the opposite of your goal.

But giving yourself the same space and freedom, to talk to other men for example, will make them take note immediately and come running back.

How does the WOSR expertly give herself the same space that a man might crave? It's pretty easy if you think about it for a second. What kind of freedom would men not want to see you with and make them feel like they don't have the upper hand anymore?

First, don't define your relationship at the first hint of ambiguity – it's that ambiguity that will drive him back to you and keep you intriguing. Once you talk about your relationship and become exclusive, you are indicating to him that you are committing to him, and eliminating even the possibility of space. Space is more beneficial because it keeps your options open and keeps you attractive.

This is positive in a general sense, but for a WOSR's pursuit of becoming attractive to a man, the space in uncertainty is important. Space retains chase and mystery. If he wanted The Talk, he would have scheduled it himself. Make him secretly beg for it and force your hand.

Chances are that if you project this air of avoiding the relationship and exclusivity talk, even if that's not what you want, he will try to change your mind. Sometimes it's not even personal at that point, but a challenge to him and his pride. He will want to close the space, and won't be happy seeing you with your own. He'll grow slightly possessive and highly interested in what you're doing with your time.

There are similar effects if you tell him you are unsure about wanting to be with him exclusively, or unsure about wanting to do long-distance... insure about wanting to date because you are coworkers... it's just going to make him want to convince you otherwise.

Second, as you have given him space in all aspects of her life... you also have space and freedom in all aspects of your life. This means in terms of talking to other men and dating them. This is really what men mean by their desire of space, so it's only fair play that you experience the same space. What follows will be eye-opening (if they are aware of the subtle hints and call-outs to your new space and lifestyle that you make public).

They'll suddenly begin checking in more with you. Randomly texting you and saying hello. Asking you to hang out more. Making time for you in their schedule. Planning a week or two ahead for you.

It's the same effect and reason that you shouldn't openly compete with other males for him — it's devaluing and shows that you can't deal with your own space.

They think you've given the space that they desire, but once they see how desirable you also are and happy you can be without them, it will drastically change his opinion on space. Such is the power of choice that you've introduced — choice is exciting, and we largely believe that all of our own choices are made for reasons we know.

So when you give him space and the freedom to select you or someone else, and they select you, they will believe that it is a genuine choice of chemistry and attraction. This is partially true — the only asterisk is that the chemistry and attraction is due to the space that you've given them that they want to fill.

You have just turned into the pursued, as he wants to close the space.

Third, people are typically intrigued by those that aren't immediately available to them. Simple human nature that has been covered, and will be covered again, in this book. Just as I was so driven and satisfied by attempting to master painting, so will the men be in trying to master you. Once you introduce space, you become painting to them – presently unattainable, but seemingly worth the effort and wait.

Finally, you must embrace the emotional and mental space from him. Do not be emotionally dependent on him, and maintain your own interests and hobbies. This is another very real void that he will begin to feel almost immediately – it will remind him of how positive and fun of an influence on his life that you have, and not allow him to use you purely as an emotional crutch, AKA the friendzone.

If they see you giving other men the duties and privileges of someone that you want to date, they will want them back immediately. Subsequently, he will feel lucky to be with you: the independent woman who has given her space, but has really just taken her own.

9. "So… What are we?"

There's always that stage when you're dating someone where you don't know what to call each other.

It's an in-between stage that causes a lot of awkwardness.

You might call them your friend, your boyfriend, look awkwardly and avoid the question, invent a label, say you're just hanging out, or avoid introducing them to your friends to avoid the topic.

Maybe you have a potential date with someone else lined up, but you don't know if that's kosher at this point – after all, if you feel guilty, isn't there something to be guilty about?

Who knows what to say? It's because you haven't talked about the terms of the relationship yet, so you don't want to slap a label on it before you know there is actually mutual interest to move forward.

I urge you to resist throwing your hands up and clearing the air with a "So… what are we?" talk for this simple reason:

Uncertainty is incredibly, incredibly arousing.

Blindfolds during sex. Anticipation before a rollercoaster. This is relationship limbo, and you get the picture. Tension remains high because every word or date could be the last.

Talking about the relationship has a few negative effects on your approach and mindset with someone, with only one real benefit – settling the uncertainty. And we all know what happens when we put someone into a corner – they immediately want their freedom. Thus, we have to make them want to put themselves in the corner voluntarily. When you don't bring up The Talk, you make it seem as if you don't want to, which will make him want to.

You want to settle the tension and uncertainty, but he feels it just as much, and it is what will drive him to you.

When he seeks subtle affirmation from you, he'll try harder to capture your attention and fish for your time. As we've seen with other subtle points in this book, this leads to him being the pursuer, and eventually actions will transform his mentality of viewing you as the desired prey. His effort will skyrocket and you will only stand to benefit.

Remaining in relationship limbo also means that he won't feel like he has a 100% hold on you. This precedes a very subtle shift in the power balance of a relationship, and can instantly shift the pants back to you if they had ever left. Have you ever heard of people growing complacent during the courting and dating phase, as opposed to the relationship phase? It just doesn't happen because there is the need to secure affection.

As always, the bitch is an expert at relationship limbo and things that generally make her appear aloof, mysterious, and attractive. She simply doesn't care enough about the man to entertain thoughts of a relationship and thus doesn't bother to confirm that with him. Moreover, she may have commitment issues and only uses men for sex instead of treating them with the respect they deserve. Finally, she may never have been in a real relationship before, period.

So how does the WOSR act in the face of relationship limbo? This chapter might embody the simplest principle in the book.

Do not bring up the future of the relationship.

You can talk about it in future terms, but only the immediate future such as next week (*Let's have brunch at that restaurant next week*). Don't talk about what you're going to do together next year. Don't be the first to refer to relationship titles and labels. Realize that your urge to settle uncertainty is damaging in the long run and only provides a small mental benefit.

Don't succumb to his pressure. Don't end up relinquishing your edge and your rightful role as the prey and pursued.

When you exit relationship limbo, you place expectations on both you and him that can be difficult to live up to. This means that you are automatically back into the role of the pursuer, because he will expect you to fulfill those expectations. And guess what – you're now expected to provide all of that, to *chase*. And this time, you are obligated to do so.

Of course, this isn't to say that committed relationships are a negative thing. The distinction that I am making is that relationship limbo can be used to jumpstart a relationship with high levels of attraction and seduction, and jumping out of relationship limbo too quickly can doom your chances.

Too many women are eager to jump into relationships when they aren't ready, or when doing so would be a turnoff to the man. So when you finally have that relationship-defining talk with him... be aware that you're not only locking yourself down.

10. How To Stay Independent And Yourself

You grew up in Rhode Island. You had tons of hobbies as a kid, and you were on the verge of pursuing dance as a professional career. You have a terrible singing voice, but you like to karaoke anyway. These days, you play in an indoor volleyball league every Tuesday, work out twice a week otherwise, and would like to train for a triathlon soon.

You've got a few college friends in the area and regularly hit up happy hours after work to socialize and unwind. One time as a child you got accidentally shaved your eyebrows, thinking that all women simply drew them in every day.

You always have a full schedule and friends have to schedule with you about one week in advance. And that's the way you like it.

Then you meet someone and it all stops.

We've all seen that scenario before, haven't we? You (or a friend) is as active and outgoing as can be, living life to the fullest, and it all suddenly disappears when they get into a relationship. Their sole focus is on spending time with their paramour, and any other priority gets dropped like a hot potato.

Their relationship has taken them hostage, and they have negotiated everything in their life for the relationship's sake. Granted, it's hard to escape in the rosy honeymoon period, and you might not even want to. But what about after the gold dust settles - where

The WOSR abides by a *no negotiation policy*.

You've worked hard to cultivate a full and fulfilling life for yourself, and really a complete identity independent of anyone else's influence or grasp. You know what you like and what do you like to do. So keep doing them! Don't negotiate your own priorities for that of the relationship (generally).

When you begin a relationship, it can be difficult to see past the rose-colored lenses of the honeymoon period. Infatuation almost dictates that you spend an inordinate amount of time together, and generally ignore all other priorities. But this is not sustainable.

If we follow that trend, you two will eventually become each other's world. You will become extremely interdependent and ultimately lose your identity. You won't be known as Cathy anymore – you'll be JimAndCathy. Whenever you go somewhere, people will just ask where your man is, and all your stories will be about him.

The WOSR does not negotiate her free time, her hobbies, her values, her ambitions, her friends, or her identity for the sake of the relationship.

Consider this a long-winded way of saying that you cannot let a man change who you are or what your priorities are. You may accommodate him, but not change yourself and your identity.

Consider how attractive the bitch is because she simply doesn't care about the man very much. She is both physically and emotionally unavailable. Whatever the case, she remains herself and doesn't kowtow to a man's schedule or demand. She will never negotiate. On a primal level, that is incredibly seductive and attractive. She projects as so high-value that you never know if you can get into her schedule so you cherish whenever you can.

Ultimately, a man likes a woman who has a strong sense of self, bitch or not. How many times have you heard a man say that he wants a woman with passions? This is the translation of that statement – please know who you are and stick to that! Men don't instantly want to become your life because that means they can't partake in their own hobbies and passions.

Here's a partial list of how the WOSR can stay true to herself:

1. Don't cancel your plans for him.
2. Form internal guidelines on how many times you see him a week.
3. No means no — you're a busy gal and shouldn't always prioritize him over your hobbies and other friends.
4. Remember that you have other friends and attempt to spend time with them accordingly.
5. No flaking (by him) is allowed — your time is precious!
6. Don't make decisions based on "I miss him" or "I just want to see him."

Having a strong sense of self with your own priorities is inherently attractive — as has been implied many times in this book. It inherently raises your value when you reduce the priority of someone else. When you're engaged, you become amazingly engaging.

If you lose that about yourself, you are essentially writing a one-way ticket to the friendzone or being a doormat. You literally will have nothing to add to the relationship other than a warm body and your presence — what about you will a man admire or even respect?

Moreover, if you were to lose yourself, what will happen if you breakup or separate? You are left with a shell of yourself, and a blinding realization that you have truly let yourself go in many ways. Few, if any friends. It's a bleak epiphany that many women reach too late.

Realize that once when you lose yourself, you are not the woman he fell in love with in the first place. You've changed, often for the worse, and men will react accordingly. It's only fair that he gets a bit disillusioned with you and moves on, because you presented him with a false image at the beginning. You've put him in a place where he has to take action or pretend to be happy.

Control over yourself – the discipline and drive to continue to pursue your interests and passions can sometimes be difficult, especially when you have to choose between them and your honey's sweet and tender embrace. But maintaining control here, and stopping the relationship terrorists, is integral to maintaining control in the relationship.

Many things are out of our hands, but if you make the sometimes difficult choice to be interesting, and not interested... then that is the key to skyrocketing attraction as a WOSR.

The obvious other hand is that there needs to be a keen balance struck between your own time, and time spent together for a healthy relationship. He does need to be a priority. But far too many women skew the other way, and are confused why their men grow bored and restless.

Look at it this way: you have a vibrant life on your own, and he is but a wonderful addition to it, though not essential. You're a new car, and you already have all your features. A man is just the power windows or sun roof.

Prioritize yourself above all else.

11. How To Never Be Taken For Granted

I have many friends that are lawyers and I believe they'll appreciate the points I'm about to make about being taken for granted.

Lawyers have a tough job.

Their very profession is in making sure that the Ts are crossed and that the Is are dotted – exact perfection is expected every single time. In fact, it's the norm. If things go well, the lawyer is never congratulated, because that means things have merely gone as planned... but if they make a small mistake, you better believe that they will have hell to pay.

They basically have one of the most thankless jobs in the world because they are taken for granted by their clients, and are only given attention when it is negative.

Where am I going with this? Lawyers are taken for granted by their clients because they are expected to produce results regardless of the situation or deadline. Unfortunately, that's in their job description.

But that description isn't included in your relationship.

Many women are taken for granted by the men they are dating because they continue to deliver regardless of the situation as if they were obligated to. They make sure they are always there regardless of the treatment they receive.

Translation: if you are doing things automatically for a man and he is expecting them automatically, you are probably being taken for granted.

When you are there with a man constantly, you are like his shadow. He will simply assume that you will always be there because... you HAVE always been there. Your actions have proven him to be right, so why should he assume any different or place any value on your presence if it is constant?

It's only when you remove something and assess the absence that you can recognize its value.

The best thing you can say about a person who is always present and taken for granted is that they are dependable... not entirely flattering, but certainly not a compelling reason to be with someone. Dependable also tends to impart a lack of excitement, allure, mystery, spontaneity, attraction... and a slew of other adjectives that make the WOSR all the more important.

The bitch, again, is a master of all things that simulate distance and indifferent to a man. She is never taken for granted because she is not there very much. Since she is not reliably there, her presence is usually a pleasant surprise like finding money in the pocket of a jacket that you haven't worn in a month.

As always, the WOSR finds a stance in the thin gray area between being a bitch and a taken for granted shadow. This is a matter of not acting in a way that lets him take you for granted, but makes him respect and cherish your time. All of his actions should prompt reactions from you, as opposed to completely catering to him, which... you got it, leads to being taken for granted.

First, predictable routines and events are the backbone of being taken for granted.

Stop them. Try to inject spontaneity and unpredictability into your relationship and life, even if you have to plan it. I should make it clear that your spontaneity should *not* include randomly surprising him with dinner and baked goods. Whatever you're doing that is automatic or routine for him, make it a special occasion or treat.

Automatic or routine things just going to further his taking you for granted, because instead of being a constant presence in his life, you are now a constant presence + acts of service or gifts, which only raises his expectations for you. You are not his mother, and it is not your duty to provide for him and perform acts of service.

Second, you are not clay.

Don't be so malleable in your priorities to make him the first and only priority on your mind. Don't cancel on other people to see him. Don't make decisions based on wanting to see him, or just wanting to hang out with him. You have other priorities and interests in your life, so indulge them!

Making personal concessions and sacrifices to spend time with him will signal that he can have his cake and eat it too... which he will expect from that point on – pretty much the definition of being taken for granted. It's not healthy, sustainable, or attractive in the slightest. Staying busy on your own terms breeds respect and desire.

Third, don't be afraid to ruffle his feathers.

Being taken for granted probably means that you are one of the most agreeable people in the world, despite the opinions you undoubtedly hold. You may not prefer to serve and always be there, but you don't feel comfortable voicing disagreement or letting people down.

You are entitled to your opinions, and entitled to get mad when someone doesn't respect them. When someone takes you for granted, they are likely steamrolling over you and not even realizing that you are the one that is compromising. When you stand up for yourself and put your foot down, it can sometimes jolt people back to appreciative reality – or at least prove a point.

Finally, observe what happens when you take away the man's boyfriend duties and give them to someone else – in essence, taking *him* for granted so much so that you don't expect anything from him. Allow someone else, male or female, to do his duties and praise them for it. He will want the duties back immediately, and for the first time feel what being taken for granted is like.

Everyone wants to feel desirable to their significant other, and part of that is direct appreciation for what they do for us.

12. How To be Confident

In a prior chapter, I begged you to act the prize and therefore become the prize. Displaying confidence and manifesting it is one of the keys to the true WOSR and cementing attraction with anyone.

This is a process that isn't the easiest for some because it can require faking it, some bravado, and acting entirely out of character at times.

This is unfortunate, as it hints strongly at a deeper issue of self-confidence and self-worth. How can you act the prize when inside you feel nothing remotely like it? The logical benefits aside, our own limiting beliefs can sometimes be the bane of our very existence. And of course, if we are limited by our own beliefs and don't have true confidence in ourselves, how can we expect others to hold us in high regard?

There are no women, whether bitch or WOSR, of either type without confidence – though it should be noted that the bitch works with insecure confidence, while the WOSR works with true confidence.

This is the pep talk chapter. The build-you-up chapter. The chapter where I convince you that you are indeed a prize, and that your confidence and actions should reflect it. Let's begin with some of my favorite quotes on confidence.

Sex appeal is fifty percent of what you've got and fifty percent what people think you've got. – Sophia Loren

To succeed in life, you need two things: ignorance and confidence. – Mark Twain

Argue for your limitations and, sure enough, they're yours. – Richard Bach

Low self-confidence isn't a life sentence. Self-confidence can be learned, practiced, and mastered – just like any other skill. Once you master it, everything in your life will change for the better. – Barrie Davenport

The way to develop self-confidence is to do the thing you fear and get a record of successful experiences behind you. – William Jennings Bryan

Don't wait until everything is just right. It will never be perfect. There will always be challenges, obstacles, and less than perfect conditions. So what. Get started now. With each step you take, you will grow stronger and stronger, more and more skilled, more and more self-confidence, and more and more successful. – Mark Victor Hansen

A few patterns emerge from the above quotes.

1. Confidence is a change that can originally stem from either outward and inward appearances. It can begin with either one, and frankly I don't think I would prefer one over the other. If you start with external changes... you will look good which will make you feel good. That mood and confidence will eventually permeate through the rest of your life. If you can revamp your physical appearance to be objectively attractive, there's no telling what you can't do!
2. A large component of confidence is the stock we put into how other people perceive us. This may not be ideal, but it's where it starts. Thus, we can take a lesson from this in observing other people's actions and assigning confidence values to them (in other words, what are the actions of a confident person versus an insecure person?). Be extremely analytical and apply those changes and suggestions to yourself.
3. On some level, any confidence you show will be irrational. It's just the nature of the beast. Even Michael Jordan, who has all the reason in the world to be confident, can sometimes be overly so and irrational. But that doesn't mean he doesn't

have a wealth of things to offer. You also do. Don't let the fear of appearing arrogant or immodest turn you off of projecting confidence, because it *will* happen. Get over that mental hurdle, and move on. You're not being presumptuous, you're just being objectively positive.

4. Once you believe you don't have confidence, you won't. Confidence starts with a belief in yourself, no matter how small. Pick one thing that you're great at – possibly the best at in the world. It can be an obscure talent that or skills, it doesn't matter how insignificant it is. We can't all be Einstein or Babe Ruth. Take pride in it, and realize you are also allowed to have those feelings of pride in things that you aren't the best at. Then compile a short list of your greatest achievements, wins, accomplishments, and otherwise feats that you would brag about. Look at it – don't you have things to be confident about?

5. Failure breeds confidence. Why? Because when you have failed, you know how badly things can go... and yet the world didn't end. Failure teaches you and lets you know just how close you were. Failures eventually turn into successes, which also breeds confidence. It's the process that is important.

6. Conditions will never be ideal for you to build confidence. It all has to start somehow and somewhere. But it's within you. That means there's never a better time than this exact moment.

7. Everyone has insecurities. But true confidence is security in who you are. Your insecurities are likely insignificant to many other people's... and it is rare that they would ever come up because everyone is so focused and self-conscious about their own. Your insecurities also add to your character because they haven't killed you yet. In that way, they actually signal that you are strong and still here. What's the realistic worst-case scenario in exposing one of your insecurities? It's probably not that bad.

Confidence can take you to your highest heights if you allow it, and it's something that you cannot compromise about yourself. Here are some actionable traits of a confident WOSR to get you started on your journey.

1. Lead others and don't be a follower
2. Don't care if others don't follow
3. Don't seek approval or affirmation from others
4. Don't be a people pleaser
5. Invest in and value yourself
6. Accept and let in the fear – it's natural

True confidence is so because of its disregard not for others, but for what others think. It's a powerful trait that is magnetic, attractive, and increasingly rare.

13. How To Make Him Feel Lucky

Enter the remora fish.

The remora fish is essentially a giant mouth with a fish body attached to it. It attaches itself to the underbelly of any sizeable shark and can remain there for its lifetime just feeding off the nutrients that the shark provides. It is a wholly unbalanced relationship in which one party is completely exploited at the expense of the other. Does this sound familiar?

Enter *Flowers for Algernon*.

Flowers for Algernon is a short novel by Daniel Keyes about a mentally retarded man who receives a surgery that turns him into a genius. He becomes incredibly self-aware, yearns for more in his life, and generally has his life enriched by the surgery. (For the purposes of this chapter, we'll ignore the part where the surgery's effects are only temporary, and he reverts back to his original mental state...)

In your relationship, are you a remora fish that only takes and doesn't give, or are you the miraculous surgery that enriches someone's life and makes them feel lucky to be alive? Moreover, is the man the remora fish or the surgery to you? The remora fish derives his or her nutrients, happiness, and fulfillment from the host – are those roles present in your relationship? Where does the balance of the relationship lie, and is there someone on the short end of the stick?

The goal for a truly healthy relationship, and one that can make marriage a not-so-scary proposition is to encourage mutual growth and development. Ideally, a couple grows and develops together, and continues to find new ways to enrich their lives. They feel lucky that they've found each other because they are both high-value, challenging individuals. This is simply not possible if either party is a remora fish.

In fact, guess what being a remora fish leads to?

You will be taken for granted.

You will become an afterthought.

You will become resented.

Worst of all, he will lose his respect for you because you wouldn't be bringing anything to the table. If you don't challenge, motivate, or inspire him, you will essentially become a body pillow. You'll have a physical presence and you'll be around to talk to him, but at best you will turn into a mere presence like a lamp.

Let's think for a moment about how the bitch challenges a man that she is dating. She probably isn't doing it on purpose. She challenges his sense of attraction by not being available or entirely interested in him. She challenges his sense of self and identity by not truly taking an interest in him and making him self-conscious and question himself. Finally, she challenges him by being not entirely nice to him, so he is forced into defensive and argumentative moods around her.

The bitch doesn't challenge and inspire so much as prod and provoke. The short term effects might be similar, but the long term effects are stunningly different.

The WOSR realizes that relationships are about bringing out the best in each other and that it takes effort and focus to do so. A relationship should be a vehicle for becoming better people – one that simultaneously supports, challenges, and inspires.

So how do you add value in such a powerful way and avoid becoming a remora fish?

It starts with yourself. The WOSR has her own expectations for herself, and it's the pursuit of fulfilling those expectations that will challenge and inspire your man. When you are engaged in many challenges, you become a challenge yourself. You increase the expectations for everything around you.

The WOSR empowers her man by cheering for him, supporting him, and asking tough questions that will help boost him to the next level whether personally or professionally. She doesn't just go through the motions when talking with him.

She frightens him sometimes because she doesn't settle.

She is a high value person, which can encourage her man to become so as well in every aspect. She takes her own professional and personal risks. She is ambitious. She works hard to cultivate a healthy relationship, and calls him out if he is not putting forth the same effort. She has little fear of failure and doesn't forego pursuing what she wants in life. She has a thirst for adventure and life in general, and doesn't accept being a couch potato with Netflix every night.

She is spontaneous and bold in her sex life and allows the man to explore his own sexuality. She doesn't avoid confrontation just for the sake of it — she realizes that the greatest growth can often come from the catharsis of challenge and resolution.

Finally, and perhaps most importantly, she truly adds value to his life in a tangible manner by leading the relationship and teaching him new things.

It all comes down to what you envision your happy relationship looking like.

Everyone has a version of the woman I described above inside them. Dig deep to find her again and reclaim your leading lady role. You are the hero of your story – are you acting it? Men don't feel lucky when they get a supporting actress.

They seek a balance of minds that contributes to mutual growth and development. Once you ensure that you yourself are challenging and inspiring, you can and should impart the rest to your partner.

14. How To Be Vulnerable

People, both men and women, simply eat up the fact that I was a near-obese infant and adolescent. Why?

Just as I had a confidence chapter earlier, this is the vulnerability chapter – arguably, the most supreme and evolved form of confidence. If confidence itself is a game-changer, consider vulnerability re-writing the rules of the game itself.

If it's not clear yet, I'm a big fan of embracing vulnerability as part of your identity and how it carries over into your relationships.

Vulnerability isn't a sob story or being a sensitive push over. When I refer to vulnerability, I mean expressing yourself without shame or apology, embracing opposition and rejection by others, and willing to take risks for your beliefs and values.

It's the principle of recognizing who you are and what you stand for, and being amazingly comfortable with it. When you're comfortable with yourself, others become comfortable with you too, and it has a certain way of putting people at ease.

Vulnerability draws others to you, and instantly makes you attractive in the sense that you are so comfortable with yourself that you can express yourself without caring about the reaction from others. It shows a sense of proactivity and introspection, as you have principles and stances based on your beliefs.

Most of all, vulnerability allows you to display supreme confidence in yourself, whether you really feel that way or not. Putting yourself out there is an admirable act, and most people will be in awe and envious of you instead of putting any judgment on you like you might think.

And that might be the root of why the bitch, true or not, is attractive. They project the air that they are content with who they are, and don't mind if you object at all. While the outwards appearance is the same, the internal intentions and principles that govern them are extremely different.

The bitch, as I've discussed before, accomplishes the veneer of vulnerability by hugely overcompensating and overstating her abilities on many things before admitting to miniscule chinks in his armor. Her ego can't survive a direct hit and unveiling of her true vulnerabilities, so she masks them with the appearance of not caring, and takes things personally later.

This leads to her attacking and lashing out at others when they open up and show their vulnerabilities because they sense an opportunity to make themselves seem more confident... at the expense of others.

I'm sure we can all name about five people off the top of our heads that partake in this.

When the WOSR truly allows vulnerability and puts a certain amount of judging power into the hands of other people, it's a powerful gesture. She doesn't have to step on anyone to maintain her confidence, and can even find the humor in his flaws and judgments that other people impose on her. People, not just men, tend to gravitate towards those that are straightforward and aren't attempting to be something they are not. They'll know what they are getting, and will in turn open up to you in a way that you ever thought possible. She's predictable, but in a positive sense.

So back to my opening statement for this chapter – why do people love the fact that I was a Michelin baby and adolescent?

It's a fact that I find hilarious about myself. Many people can often relate to it. It disarms people and shows that I don't take myself that seriously. It shows that I have no issues letting chinks like that slide, and that I don't care if they tend to diminish my overall image. Most of all, I'm confident enough in myself to turn something potentially embarrassing into a uniquely vulnerable connecting point.

I am who I am, and you can accept me or not. And more often than not, after I share it, I get back something that they are insecure about or that makes them vulnerable, and an instant deep bond is created.

Let's look at the other side:

If I was to be ashamed of this small fact, how would it reflect on the rest of my self-image and how others could deal with it? They would know that it's a sore spot, and would have to avoid it altogether. Tensions rise, and must be diverted.

A WOSR's ability to be the attractive woman that a man desires in a relationship is directly proportional to how vulnerable she is willing to make himself. Vulnerability is what communicates a woman's desires, and if they are actually expressed.

The flip side, of course, is the doormat who can only claim ownership to the pants of a relationship once in a blue moon. She doesn't freely express her opinion, is a pushover, and seeks to please people (in this case, the man of the relationship) instead of live her own life.

The doormat is mired in her label because she doesn't make himself vulnerable – she's simply not willing to take the leap of attempting to assert herself or open herself up to judgment in any way. What then is interesting or attractive to the man in the long term?

Vulnerability is an often overlooked element of attraction and self-esteem. Of course, even though I've told you how people subconsciously embrace the presence of vulnerability and impart a slew of positive adjectives to it, it doesn't mean that you won't have your mental blocks preventing you from immediately telling people your business.

Vulnerability is a process, but is one well-worthy of conquering as the pinnacle of confidence.

Conclusion

Now who can tell me the difference between a WOSR and a bitch?

Here's the version I've been hopefully imparting throughout the book: we are attracted to confidence, independence, and challenge. The bitch manifests these attractive features and traits because she simply doesn't care about the men she sees. Distance, apathy, and a lack of prioritization are, strangely enough, similar enough externally to be perceived as strength.

On the flip side, the WOSR is attractive because even though she actually cares about the men she sees, she is truly confident and independent as a result of her lifestyle and prioritization of herself.

Here's the final summary for this book: the bitch is attractive because she puts up a front, while the WOSR is attractive because she doesn't *have to* front.

I hope you realize the powerful lesson herein that you can remain your true self – the sweet girl, the caring girl, the girl who men will want to take home to their mothers immediately – and yet attract men with the biggest and baddest bitches out there. If you follow my tenets within, you'll have truly impacted your entire life and upgraded yourself in every way imaginable.

The WOSR is a mindset and a lifestyle that, just by gaining awareness of it, can skyrocket you into the stratosphere and help you conquer goals you never thought possible.

Men *want* to love women like you, and you now have the tools to step up and announce your presence to them.

Finish last? This sweet girl never will again.

Sincerely,

Patrick King
www.PatrickKingConsulting.com

P.S. If you enjoyed this book, I would really appreciate if you left me a review on Amazon!

The WOSR Cheat Sheet

1. How To Never Chase

If you chase too much, too openly, too obviously, or too strongly, your pursuit will make him run from you like a gazelle. There's nothing attractive about being pursued so single-mindedly, and will lead to him devaluing you. Turn the tables and make him chase you.

2. How to Create a Vacuum for Pursuit

When you pull away, you create a vacuum that he will immediately want to fill... a process that turns him into the pursuer and can change the perception of the relationship's dynamics completely.

3. How To Not Cling

Maintain your independence from a man, because if you start becoming dependent on him, you've robbed him of his own independence and given him total control… both of which are justified grounds for getting bored and losing respect for you. You've changed from the woman who attracted him in the first place, so no wonder.

4. How To Never Be A Doormat

Your partner wants an equal and someone they can go toe-to-toe with. Prioritize your own interests and hobbies and don't make decisions based simply on wanting to spend time with him. You are not defined by him or the relationship; you weren't before you met him, so you shouldn't change after.

5. How To Use Anticipation

Anticipation and the lack of certainty is an incredible aphrodisiac and will draw men to you. Prolong the "chase" by simply being a busy person, and not artificially manipulating your availability.

6. How To Be The Prize

When you perceive yourself as a high-value person, you act like it, and everyone else will follow your lead. Don't accept when others treat you like a backup or otherwise, because that will snowball.

7. Not To Not Mother And Nag

A mother nags, dotes, and is a general nuisance that makes her son want space and separation. A mate takes care of her man, but does so in a way that is more primal, subtle, and only creates more attraction.

8. How To Seize Your Own Space

When you give a man space, who knows what he'll do with it. However, when you take the same space that he might want from you, and he notices, he will likely regret her choice immediately and want to close that space.

9. "So... What are we?"

Resist the urge to define and spell out your feelings on where you want or see your relationship going until it is absolutely necessary. Again, uncertainty builds sexual tension, desire, and wanting.

10. How To Stay Independent And Yourself

Prioritize yourself and don't negotiate your own values or interests for the good of a relationship. Maintain a strong sense of self because when you are engaged, you become engaging.

11. How To Never Be Taken For Granted

Do not act in a way that enables others to take you for granted, and react appropriately when they do. Don't be afraid to make waves or assert yourself. Don't get into the habit of letting him expect acts from you automatically.

12. How To Be Confident

True confidence stems from being comfortable with your flaws and the realization that no one cares about them because they are too consumed with their own.

13. How To Make Him Feel Lucky

Don't be a remora fish. Add value to his life by ensuring that you are challenging and inspiring yourself – and he will follow suit.

14. How To Be Vulnerable

When you're comfortable with your vulnerabilities and flaws, it puts others at ease and makes them open up to you in ways you never thought possible. Vulnerability is also the height of real confidence.

www.ingramcontent.com/pod-product-compliance
Lightning Source LLC
Chambersburg PA
CBHW062050280526
45788CB00003B/1172